# LIPOI

# REMOVAL

## A COMPREHENSIVE GUIDE
## AND TOOLKIT FOR LIPOMA TREATMENT

# Thomas K. McPherson

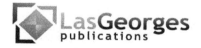

LasGeorges
publications

United Kingdom

# LIPOMA REMOVAL GUIDE

Copyright © LasGEORGES Publications 2013
www.LasGeorgesPublications.com

LasGEORGES Publications has asserted the right under the Copyright Designs and Patent Act 1988 to be the owner of this work.

Cover Designed by Dr. Jay Polma

A CIP catalogue record of this book is available from the British Library.

ISBN 978-0-9575791-1-8

Thomas McPherson

# Contents

*Introduction* ............................................................. xiii

**Lipoma Explained** ................................................... 1

How Common is Lipoma? ...................................... 2

Current Statistical Data ........................................... 3

**Different Types of Lipoma** ................................... 5

AngioLipoma or Underlying Lipoma ..................... 7

Superficial Subcutaneous Lipoma .......................... 7

Neural Fibro Lipoma ............................................. 10

Chondroid Lipoma ................................................ 11

Myelolipoma .......................................................... 12

Spindle Cell Lipoma .............................................. 12

Pleomorphic lipomas ............................................. 13

Fibrolipoma ........................................................... 13

Painful Lipoma ...................................................... 14

Facial Lipoma ........................................................ 15

Breast Lipoma ........................................................ 16

Belly Lipoma ........................................................ 17

Intramuscular Lipoma.......................................... 18

Colon Lipoma ...................................................... 19

**Dercum's disease** ................................................ 21

The Symptoms of Adiposis Dolorosa.................... 22

Prevalence of adiposis dolorosa .......................... 23

Causes of Adiposis Dolorosa................................ 23

**Lipoma in dogs and birds**.................................... 25

Lipoma in dogs .................................................... 25

Lipoma In Birds.................................................... 29

**What Causes Lipoma in Human**.......................... 33

Diet? .................................................................... 34

Genetic factors? .................................................. 35

**Symptoms of Lipoma**.......................................... 39

Early signs............................................................ 39

Classifying the Stages of Lipoma.......................... 40

Common Features of Lipoma ................................ 41

**Diagnosis of lipoma** ............................................ 43

Physical examination............................................ 43

Radiological Imaging............................................ 44

Laboratory examination ............................................. 44

Diagnosis Through Biopsy ........................................ 45

Self-Assessment at Home .......................................... 46

Common Misdiagnosis for Lipoma............................. 47

Lipoma Undiagnosed Conditions.............................. 48

Why Lipomas Are Often Undiagnosed ..................... 48

**Exploring Specific Causes** ...................................... 51

Prevalence and Common Risk Factors....................... 51

**Lipoma Treatment**................................................. 55

Treatment Options .................................................. 55

Conventional Treatment Methods to remove Lipoma. 56

Alternative Solutions For Lipoma .............................. 66

**Non-Surgical and Alternative Methods** ..................... 69

Detoxification Recipes .............................................. 70

Acupuncture In Lipoma Treatment ............................ 74

Natural and Home Remedies ..................................... 75

**Physical Exercise Approach to Lipoma removal** ....... 85

Factors Leading To Overweight.................................. 86

Dieting and Lipoma................................................. 89

**Managing Lipoma: Helpful Tips**................................ 93

Living with a Person with Lipoma .................................. 93

Aids for People with Lipoma .......................................... 94

**Concluding Remarks** ..................................................... 97

A More Serious Problem ................................................. 97

Complications Due To Lipoma ........................................ 98

Treating Lipoma To Avoid Complications ................... 98

Lipoma and Self Esteem .................................................. 99

Chronic Inflammation in the Body .............................. 100

Lipoma And Medications For HIV .............................. 102

Lipoma Treatment and Insurance Coverage ............... 103

**Lipoma FAQ** ................................................................. 105

**Useful Websites** ........................................................... 111

USA – ................................................................................ 111

Websites offering liposuctions in US, Canada, Australia
& UK ................................................................................ 112

Canada ............................................................................. 113

Australia ........................................................................... 114

United Kingdom ............................................................. 115

*References* ...................................................................... 117

*Index* ................................................................................ 121

*This detailed, well-researched, comprehensive treatment guide and toolkit is dedicated to all lipoma sufferers all over the world.*

## "I just wish I had found this book earlier"

"For the past 13 years I have suffered from many lipo-mas and painless but disgusting fatty lumps all over my body including my face. I am so grateful that I came across this awesome information. So practical and effective, it is still hard to believe, so many people including health professionals take into the conven-tional approach that does nothing but put patches on fatty lumps for a while, only to grow back with a vengeance. I just wish I had found this book earlier. It would have saved me a lot of expenses and misery. This book is a miracle"

## Claire Billet. *London UK*

# Introduction

Just imagine you woke up one morning to find a soft mass of fatty tissue bulging out from under your skin's surface. This growth is not painful. In fact, it has been growing slowly and steadily over a period. Could it be a cancerous growth? That is not necessarily so – this fatty growth is a Lipoma.

You usually find these soft, fatty masses in areas which are prone to cellulite. That is why you may find them underneath your elbows, at the back of your thighs, neck, arms, and back.

You will find this book to be one of the best volumes providing detailed information on Lipoma. It contains everything you need to know about Lipoma including but not limited to causes, symptoms, diagnosis, proven and most effective treatment methods, and the online resources, where you can use to obtain more information.

# CHAPTER 1

# Lipoma Explained

Lipoma is a common skin disorder affecting millions of people around the world today. It is a non-cancerous or benign skin tumor that can appear and grow in different parts of the body. Lipoma can be determined through the lumps that grow just under the skin. These lumps contain fatty cells and usually move when pressed by the fingers. Most fatty lumps are not painful even when pinched, making lipomas unnoticed for years before it can be diagnosed.

Lipomas are benign, non-cancerous, harmless and most of the time painless growth of fatty tissue just right behind or under the skin. The growth of lipoma is slow, and you would not even know that you have a lipoma for several years unless you can clearly see the bulge in your skin. This medical condition can happen to anyone at any age, but most cases of lipomas are commonly found from individuals aging from 40 to 60 years old. Moreover, lipoma is more common to men than women. There are different names or types of lipomas depending on the area of growth and the composition of the tumor. We will discuss the type later.

Despite many painstaking researches and studies about this skin condition, there are no consensus on its causes yet, making it difficult to determine the actual ways to prevent it. Lipomas can also occur in dogs, but just like in human lipomas, no known causes are also proven and accepted by the medical experts.

---

## How Common is Lipoma?

Lipoma affects millions around the world.

Women, especially in the age group of 30 to 40 are more prone to common single Lipoma. Nevertheless, there are no hard and fast rules about Lipoma being prevalent in one age group, gender or race.

If you are genetically predisposed to Lipoma or you have members in your family suffering from cancer, you may also find this growth, sometime during your life.

> Men in the age group of 40 – 60 may be more prone to Lipomatosis, which is a condition related to multiple Lipoma lumpy growths on the neck, shoulders, back and legs.

## Current Statistical Data

According to a survey conducted online where online visitors who experienced or suffer from the condition can join, only few patients or about 30% of the total participants have undergone surgery to remove their lipomas. However, from the online participants, 23% of the patients who participated reported that their lipomas grew back after the surgery.

Based on the patients' reports, most of the lipomas were found in the upper leg or thighs to the knee, in the lower arm, and in the upper arm. Some lipomas were also found in the back, in the abdomen, in the chest area, and in the lower leg. Some few lumps were reported to have been found in the shoulder, underarm, in the neck, hands, and few on the face.

Most of the patients who have lipomas preferred dermatologists to help with their problem. Some also go to a general physician while some go to a plastic surgeon especially for patients who preferred to undergo excision surgery for the removal of their lipomas.

Although surgeries and treatments are available, most physicians or dermatologists do not immediately recommend these options unless the lipomas affect the person's appearance like those lumps growing on the face or for lipomas that are causing pain due to their sensitive position. Some lipomas may unluckily grow in a dangerous or complicated area of the body like near the spine, near a vital organ, or the air passage affecting the person's proper breathing. When lipomas appear in these sensitive areas of the body, then excision of lipoma might be advised by the doctor in order to prevent complications.

Lipomas may also be necessarily removed due to the growing lumps, which may hit crucial parts of the body like nerves or blood vessels. When the growing benign lumps pinch nerves or blood vessels, it can cause pain and inflammation to the pinched nerves that in return may affect a person's mobility and functioning.

# CHAPTER 2

# Different Types of Lipoma

It is also necessary to understand the different types of lipomas. According to health experts, there are different types of lipomas that can grow in the body and some of the most common are superficial subcutaneous lipoma, spindle cell lipoma, hibernoma, pleomorhpic lipoma, and chondroid lipoma.

Superficial subcutaneous lipoma is the most common type of lipoma today and usually appears in the thighs, torsos, and forearms. They also usually appear in areas of the body that has fats. Spindle cell lipoma is a slow growing benign tumor that usually occurs in males. They are commonly found in the neck, shoulders, and posterior back of elderly males.

Lipoma tends to share a lot of common symptoms to other health conditions especially serious diseases like skin cancer and breast cancer. To prevent misdiagnosis of lipoma, proper tests may be required such as physical exams and biopsy or extraction of tissue samples for laboratory examination aside from the common imaging tests mentioned above like MRI and CT scan.

Proper knowledge about the condition is also vital in order to be prepared if you have lumps growing under the skin in various parts of your body. Immediately consult a doctor or much better, a dermatologist so you can get the right treatments in case you have a more serious condition other than lipoma.

Lipomas are usually named based on the location they have developed. Lipomas are benign tumors that usually contain fibrous tissue, vascular structures, and fatty tissues with collagen. They are usually inherited but are sometimes caused by tissue injury or trauma. Anyone who has these soft tissue tumors does not necessarily need medication or treatment. Surgery or medication is only needed when this medical condition compresses organs or nerve tissues, which brought discomfort to the person.

There are many types of lipomas and the most common ones are formed beneath the skin. The bulging mass beneath the skin is usually movable beneath the skin surface when pressed by fingers. This is the most common growth of lipomas and contains adipose tissue which is surrounded by a fibrous outer covering. The size of lipomas usually ranges from 2.54 centimeters or fewer.

# AngioLipoma or Underlying Lipoma

Angiolipomas usually develop in the young adults and mostly have multiple growths in the chest and arms of a person. This tumor got its name from its' contains which includes complex vascular structures and adipose or fatty tissues. These tumors usually requires a surgery because patients from this type of medical condition usually complain of pain and discomfort.

# Superficial Subcutaneous Lipoma

This is the most common or conventional for of lipomas. This lies just underneath the skin and can be found mainly in the forearms, thighs and trunks. They can also grow anywhere in the body where body fat is located.

## Lumbosacral Lipoma

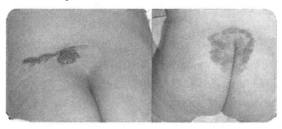

This lipoma usually appears on the back of infants. However, it can also affect adults.

## Diffuse Lipomatosis

This is a rare type of Lipoma, which normally affects babies up to the age of two. These lipomas may be superficial, or they may be deep-seated. They cover the body extensively in multiple lumps.

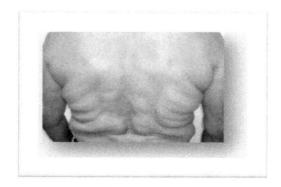

## Angiolipoma

Angliolipoma is also a type of lipoma that usually develops or shows as multiple growths on the chest and arms of the young adults. This lipoma derived its name from its components, which is a combination of adipose tissue or fatty acids and complex vascular structures. Individuals suffering from angliolipomas usually complain about the discomfort it brings.

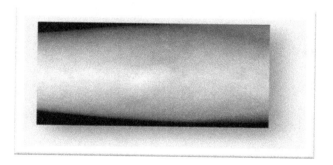

This is the rare lipoma, normally found in muscle cells, blood vessels, connective tissue and fatty tissue.

## Intradermal Spindle Cell Lipoma

This is commonly found in women, growing on the back, shoulders and neck area.

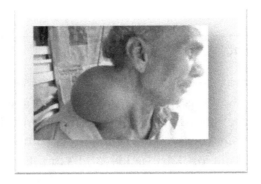

---

*Pleomorphic Lipoma or Fatty Lipoma*

This is usually found in the elderly. One of the side effects of this Lipoma is joint pain.

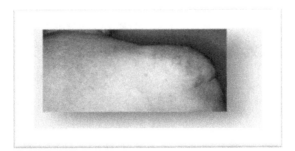

---

# Neural Fibro Lipoma

This Lipoma exerts pressure on nerves, due to its growth. This gives rise to the condition Adiposis Dolorosa.

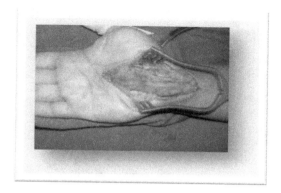

## Chondroid Lipoma

Although lipomas are more common in men, women can also have a lipoma. Chondroid lipoma is common among women and usually occurs in the leg area. Knowing these different types of lipoma will give you an idea of your current condition. By doing so, you can make a good decision that is beneficial for your health.

Here, this yellow colored fatty tumor grows on the lower extremities of your body or the neck.

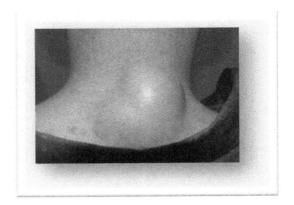

## Myelolipoma

Myelolipoma is the uncommon form of lipoma. This tumor is composed of fatty tissues, and red and white cells. It inhibits platelets-forming abilities just like the bone marrows. This type of tumor can be found or usually develops inside or outside the adrenal gland. Myelolipomas can be found most often in men aging from 40 to 60 years old. Individuals under this medical condition experience hypertension, pain from organ compression, and blood urine.

## Spindle Cell Lipoma

Spindle cell lipomas are often mistaken as a malignant liposarcoma. This lipoma is firmer when touched as compared to the normal lipoma masses. Spindle cell lipomas contain yellow, white and gray coloration. It consists of spindle-shaped cells, mucus material and bundles of fibrous tissues. This lipoma usually affects males aging from 45 up to 70.

## Pleomorphic lipomas

Pleomorphic lipomas can usually be found at the back of the neck, shoulders and upper back. Unlike the normal lipomas, this lipoma varies in the fat content, which is ranging from 10% up to 90%. Along with the fat contents, it is also composed of blood vessels, empty spaces, and bundles of collagen fibers.

## Fibrolipoma

Fibrolipoma is another lipoma which may develop anywhere in the human body and is composed of a mixture of fibrous tissues and fatty acids. However, most of the cases of Fibrolipomas are found inside and around the area of the mouth and in the gastrointestinal tract. Fibrolipomas are often the cause of nerve compression, lymphedema and are sometimes associated to hemorrhage.

# Painful Lipoma

Most lipomas are not painful making them hard to diagnose at its early stage. They can grow unnoticed for years since they tend to grow slow especially when they appear in hidden or unexposed areas of the body. However, some lipomas may be painful if they are located in delicate areas of the body. Some lumps become painful because they hurt or pinch nerves or blood vessels. Lipomas can also lead to difficulty in breathing if they appear near or within the air passages for breathing.

Some lumps can also be dangerous if they appear near vital organs, near the spine, and grow large. However, these cases are usually extremely rare. Infection is also possible making the lumps painful to touch and may also lead to foul-smelling discharges directly from the lumps.

If you have lipoma and the fatty lumps become tender and painful to touch, then it is time to consider treatment or removal of lipoma to avoid complications and also to avoid the condition from affecting your movement and daily functioning.

> One of the immediate reliefs for pain caused by fatty lumps under the skin would be immediate removal of the tumors. Most physicians do not recommend excision surgeries for lipomas, but once the tumors became infected or painful, treatments and possible surgeries may be recommended to prevent complications and provide relief from the pain.

However, if you do not want to resort to invasive procedures like excision of lipoma, you can also opt for a milder option like steroid injection. Injection for lipoma can also provide relief from the pain since steroid injections effectively shrink the fatty lumps under the skin.

## Facial Lipoma

A facial Lipoma is rather rare, but it has been known to occur. You may find a painless tumor growing on some parts of your face and soon this lump which is fatty, soft and spongy in texture may start to look really visible. Facial Lipomas are definitely not good to look at and that is why it is necessary that you meet your doctor as soon as possible and asking for the best treatment.

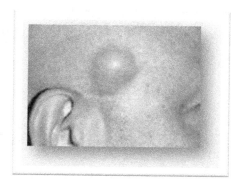

# Breast Lipoma

A breast Lipoma is a noncancerous fatty fleshy growth growing under the surface of the skin on your breasts. These Lipomas may be hereditary or they may have been caused due to some trauma to the breast tissue.

Breast Lipomas normally occur when fatty cells start to proliferate at an abnormal rate, causing a soft lumpy mass of tissue. This is painless and keeps moving around under the surface of the skin.

Women are more prone to breast Lipomas, especially if they are genetically prone to this condition. These Lipomas when removed surgically resemble the yellow fat masses normally found in poultry, under the skin.

The size of a breast Lipoma can be anywhere between 1 to 4 centimeters in diameter. Regular monitoring needs to be done to check its growth and condition.

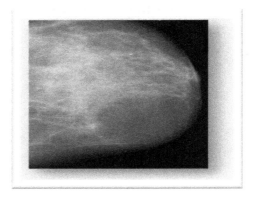

Looking for lumps on one's breast region is one of the usual self check health procedures done by health-conscious women at home. This is to check whether there is any cancerous growth on the breasts.

Cancerous tissue is normally going to show up as hard lumps which need to be checked and tested in the laboratory. In the same manner, Lipomas are also slow growing, painless and soft, spongy tumors, which can grow anywhere on your body, including on your belly. Just palpate this mass with your fingers.

You can feel this moving pulpy mass as just one lump or a number of lumps, anywhere between 1 to 3 centimeters in size.

## Belly Lipoma

A belly Lipoma is going to protrude from under the surface of your skin. It is normally going to be found in areas where there are fatty deposits already present, especially around the waist or in the chest region. Surgical removal is recommended for getting rid of these unsightly belly Lipomas.

## Intramuscular Lipoma

There are two types of Lipomas which are connected to the muscles. Intramuscular Lipomas normally grow inside the muscle tissue. This is fatty tissue, which grows inside the muscles in the legs, head, neck, shoulder region and body of adults.

As this is not a life-threatening condition, doctors will not normally recommend surgical removal unless the Lipoma begins to grow really fast, or is the cause of Adiposis Dolorosa.

Also, intramuscular Lipoma surgery is a very intricate procedure, because this fatty deposit is deep-seated and connected to the muscles. A doctor does not want to take the chance of cutting through muscles to prevent further complications)

Intramuscular lipomas normally affect men in the 30 to 60 age group. The large muscles of the legs are the most commonly affected portions of the body during this condition.

In the same manner, the second type of muscle related lipomas, known as intramuscular Lipomas grow between a group of muscles. This sort of Lipoma can be removed easily through surgical procedures.

The recovery time of the patient after such surgical procedures is anywhere between 1 to 3 days, depending on the size and location of the inter-muscular Lipoma. There is also the possible side effect of the tumor growth recurring again because of incomplete removal of the Lipoma does happen in one percent of the cases.

---

## Colon Lipoma

A Lipoma growth can occur anywhere on your body, especially if you are genetically prone to it. That means that Lipoma growth have been known to occur on the colon and even on other internal organs of the body.

Such a Lipoma is asymptomatic and may be found just by chance during a colonoscopy or during a surgical procedure. Colon Lipomas have a higher occurrence in women, especially women in their 60s. A colon Lipoma is benign fatty tumors, which can be anywhere between some millimeters to 40 centimeters in size. Some patients may feel vague symptoms like stomach pain and change in normal bowel habits when suffering from Colon Lipomas.

Doctors may remove colon Lipomas by endoscopic surgical procedures. A colon Lipoma is diagnosed with the help of Endoscopic Ultrasound [EUS.]

Lipomas in this particular region may cause gastrointestinal bleeding, as well as obstruction in the digestive tract. The bleeding is caused due to ulceration. That is why even though this tumor is a benign mass, it is considered to be malignant, because of its position and location.

# CHAPTER 3

# Dercum's disease

## Adiposis Dolorosa, known as Dercum's Disease

This is a condition characterized by multiple painful fatty swellings and most commonly affects postmenstrual women who are obese. The patients suffering from this type of lipoma usually describe it as "all the fat hurts" and it increases with the increase in the fatty tissue. In patients suffering from the adiposis dolorosa disease, the lipomas usually occur anywhere on the body though most often found on upper parts of the arms, legs, buttocks, and torso.

Although it is a rare disease, adiposis dolorosa is the most painful type of lipoma. The lipomas cause burning or severe aching; the pain can come and go or can be continuous.

## The Symptoms of Adiposis Dolorosa

The signs and symptoms of adiposis Dolorosa typically appear between the ages 35 and 50 and include the following:

Painful skin lumps

Reduced sweating

Absence of menstruation

Headache

Asthenia

Bruises

Reduced skin sensitivity

Painful fatty skin lumps

General Weakness and tiredness

Epilepsy

Dementia

Irritability

Mental disturbances

Asthenia

fatigability

## Prevalence of adiposis dolorosa

This type of lipoma is known as a rare disease whose prevalence is unknown. Bases on unclear reasons, adiposis dolorosa occur in women up to 30 times more often than in men.

## Causes of Adiposis Dolorosa

The causes of adiposis dolorosa are poorly researched and no one knows them. Due to the discomfort associated with this condition, many patients are unable to fully perform normal activities of daily living. The disorder can grow slowly over many years or rapidly due to external stress like flu, pregnancy, or surgery. Dercum disease (adiposis dolorosa) is believed to be inherited in an autosomal dominant way. Most specifically is believed to be transmitted in the line of great grandmother-mother-daughter.

No known genes associated to the adiposis dolorosa have been identified. There are several probable causes of this condition that have been suggested but none have been confirmed. Some of the suggested causes include the use of corticosteroids, breakdown of fat and changes in deposition, as well as dysfunction of the endocrine system.

### *What other names are usually used for adiposis dolorosA?*

morbus Dercum

lipomatosis dolorosa

Dercum-Vitaut syndrome

Dercum's disease

Dercum disease

Anders syndrome

adipose tissue rheumatism

adiposalgia

# CHAPTER 4

# Lipoma in dogs and birds

## Lipoma in dogs

Did you know that Lipoma is not restricted to just human beings? Dogs can also suffer from this condition. If you keep dog and your dog is overweight from lack of physical exercise, there is a chance that she may suffer from Lipoma especially when she is growing older.

Many dog owners get really anxious whenever they see this soft fatty tumor showing up on their well-loved pets.

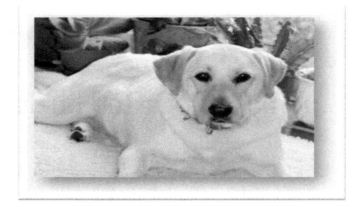

You do not need to worry unless your dog is suffering any discomfort. It is only in such cases that the vet is going to recommend the Lipoma be removed. Remember that any sort of tumor growth is not a healthy sign in humans or in canines. So if you see a possible Lipoma on your old dog, contact the vet immediately so that he can diagnose the condition.

## Sites of lipoma in dogs

You normally see this Lipoma mass on your dog's underbelly, chest region and abdomen. Lipoma in dogs may look unsightly, but it is not life-threatening. Old Labrador Retrievers, Doberman Pinschers and other small and medium-size dog breeds are more vulnerable to canine Lipoma.

Your vet may recommend a biopsy to diagnose the status of this fatty lump. He is then going to give you the best advice. A surgical removal is necessary only if the Lipoma shows abnormal growth and starts to cause the dog discomfort during movement, or any other activity.

So the moment you see a Lipoma on your pet dog, talk to the vet for proper advice, diagnosis, and necessary treatment.

## Causes of Lipoma In Dogs

Lipomas can be found in dogs especially those that are obese and old. Despite various studies about this condition, there are no known or confirmed causes of lipomas in dogs yet. This is why there are also no solid preventive measures available yet in order to fight and prevent lipomas in dogs.

### Obesity in Dogs

As mentioned above, there are no sufficient evidences yet that would prove or point the specific causes of lipoma in dogs. However, a lot of theories are available and considered as guide by veterinarians and dog health experts. Because most of the dogs with lipomas are quite overweight or obese, one of the theorized probable causes of lipoma is obesity that is connected with their diet.

Most dog experts believe that diets of dogs can affect or increase the probably of acquiring lipoma in dogs.

Lipomas itself are fatty lumps or cysts under the skin and dogs who commonly eat foods rich in fats and carbohydrates are believed to be at higher risks of getting this condition.

## Hormonal Problems In Dogs

Hormonal problem is another speculated cause of lipoma in dogs as well as in humans. According to some studies, the fatty lumps may have been caused by intensive hormonal activities causing imbalance to the dog's hormonal state. These hormonal imbalances may also be caused by a specific underlying condition or problem in the dog's body and health or may be caused by a specific situation the dog is experiencing like pregnancy. This is why lipomas are also more common in female dogs than in male. Medications or specific types of drugs given to dogs may also cause hormonal imbalance.

## Heredity and Old Age

Since most lipomas are detected during the middle age, some dog experts believe that lipomas can be caused by aging or it can also be a hereditary condition since there are some specific dog breeds that are more prone to lipomas such as the dachshunds, cocker spaniels, terriers, and poodles. However, lipomas are also found in other dog breeds although in minimal cases so make sure to watch out for lumps and always check the skin of your dogs when you have one.

Just like in humans, lipomas are benign tumors so they are not that dangerous. Most veterinarians do not recommend treatments or surgical removal procedures when dogs have lipomas in areas that do not cause pain or affect movements.

Most surgical removal of lipomas in dogs is advised when the lipomas are situated in the area that causes pain or it affects the movement and the functioning of the dogs. Some lipomas may also cause itchiness causing your dog to always scratch and chew the affected area, which may then result to infection and inflammation. When these complications occur, make sure to immediately consult your dog vet to get the proper treatment for your dog's condition.

Because of the idea that lipomas are non-cancerous, some dog owners generalize all fatty lumps in the dog as lipomas. When your dog have many lumps growing around the body, make sure to have it checked by a veterinarian to make sure that none of it is cancerous or life threatening.

## Lipoma In Birds

Avian lipoma is a benign skin disease that leads to the formation of fatty lumps underneath the bird's skin. Just like in lipomas in humans and dogs, avian lipomas are also noncancerous but lipomas in birds are more prone to complication due to the small and delicate body of the birds, and their tendencies to pick the affected area resulting to infection and bleeding.

Most of the fatty lumps in birds occur in the stomach and in the chest but avian lipoma can also appear in other areas of the body, even internally. Lipomas birds can also vary in size. Some avian lipomas are very small while some may be big in size enough to affect the bird's mobility and functions. The most dangerous aspect of having avian lipoma is that the birds tend to pick the affected area which may then lead to bleeding, necrotic tumors, and worst, death.

---

## Main Causes Of Lipomas In Birds

### Excess Weight or Obesity

One of the common causes of lipomas in birds is obesity or being overweight. The excess weight can be caused by dietary factors like feeding birds with foods high in fat content or deficiency in Vitamin E leading to poor metabolism. Birds have the tendency to store excess fats as part of their body's mechanism. However, too much deposit can build up if the bird is eating too much fatty foods or when metabolism is too slow resulting to build up of excess fats in the liver and in other tissues of the body.

## Genetic Predisposition

Genetics is also another common cause of avian lipoma. All birds can be affected by this benign tumor especially those with unhealthy and fatty diets. However, some varieties of birds tend to often get this condition despite being healthy and active. Some species of birds that are prone to avian lipoma are budgies or budgerigars, galahs, Amazons, rosellas, and sulphur crested cockatoos.

If your bird is quite active, not overweight, and you feed it with healthy less-fatty foods, then the tumor must most likely have been triggered by genetic predisposition. For birds that are prone to avian lipoma due to genetic, well-balanced diet and exercise are definitely important to prevent the occurrence of lipoma or to prevent the lumps from growing.

## Hypothyroidism

Hypothyroidism in birds is also another factor for the development of lipoma in birds. This condition is usually caused by lack of iron in the body. Hypothyroidism can lead to inflammatory skin diseases and traumatic dermatitis like lipoma.

Most lipomas in birds are not that dangerous and can be treated through improved diet, increased exercise, and iodine supplements. However, some avian lipomas can develop into more dangerous conditions like Xanthoma, this is when lipomas become necrotic or ulcerated, and can lead to bleeding episodes leading to death.

When lipomas progress to Xanthoma, immediate surgery to remove the infected lumps may be recommended by veterinarians. Laser therapy can also be advised to reduce the size of the lumps and to provide immediate relief for the birds without the need for surgery.

# CHAPTER 5

# What Causes Lipoma in Human

Lipoma is not yet fully understood in terms of its causes. Some believe that lipomas are caused by genetics or heredity and can be triggered by minor injuries. There are cases where several of the family members have lipomas at the same time. This idea bothers many people especially for those who have parents that got the lipoma tumor, greater chances that they may also get the same condition in their lifetime. Further research in the field of medicine is still required in order to fully understand the origin, cause and other details regarding lipomas.

There are cases where lipomas develop after an injury or accident. For example, a solid blow to the body or in cases when our body tissue suffers from a trauma can also trigger lipomas.

Another perspective about the cause of lipomas is poor or unhealthy nutrition, insufficient exercise and unhealthy lifestyle. The improper activities and lifestyle have also be suggested as one of the cause of the tumors in our body.

## Diet?

Some experts believe that Lipomas may be triggered off through your diet. In fact, a body which has not undergone systematic detoxification and has a huge toxin buildup may be more prone to Lipomas. That is because the liver is finding it difficult to break down the toxins which have a nasty long-term effect on the general health of your body.

Some medical experts suggest a change in lifestyle and diet, especially adding more fruits and vegetables to your diet. Whether this influences the growth of Lipomas or not this factor is going to have a positive effect on your general health. That is why a good and healthy nutritional diet may prevent Lipomas from occurring.

It has been noticed that chemical preservatives in your food do plenty of harm to your health in the long run. That is why it is advisable to reduce dietary food items with plenty of chemical preservatives in them. Also try to reduce tobacco and alcohol abuse.

Proper detoxification of your body at regular intervals is a good way in which you can get rid of toxins. Accumulated Toxins may be one of the reasons why a tumor growth of fatty cells has taken place in your body. Try this diet, and change in lifestyle –Reduce foodstuffs in your diet, which are hard to digest. These include a high-protein diet, like meat, fat, and dairy products. Instead, start to concentrate on omega 3 rich foods like fish, cereals, fruit, fresh vegetables, whole grains, seeds and nuts.

This is going to have a beneficial long-term effect on your health. It also means that you are not going to put on extra fat. As lipomas are normally present in areas with high fat content, this can reduce the possibility of a future Lipoma growth. You can also increase your intake of health supplements and vitamins, if you do not get the proper essential nutrients in your normal daily diet. These nutrients include vitamins, minerals, necessary carbohydrates and proteins and a little fat to keep your body functioning properly and in a healthy manner.

## Genetic factors?

Although there are no exact causes of lipoma, a lot of health experts propose theories and studies about the possible causes of this benign skin condition and one of the most popular and widely accepted theory is genetics and hereditary. According to medical experts, lipoma can occur by inheritance since most lipomas appear in members of the family or even in relatives.

Based on a study on lipomas conducted in 1993, most of the patients with lipomas that participated in the study reported that one of their parents also has the skin condition, adding to the anecdotal evidence that lipoma can be really passed from generation to generation.

If one of your parents has lipoma or even some distant relatives have this condition, it is important to eat proper foods and maintain a healthy lifestyle in order to reduce the risk of acquiring the skin disease. Although there are no specific studies that would prove the lipoma can be caused by obesity since lipomas are composed of fatty soft tissues, some health experts recommend that people with the condition or at risk, should regularly drink lemon juice.

Lemon juice is a popular fruit known to have detoxifying properties, which effectively eliminate toxins in the body as well as fat deposits in the skin, and also boost digestion of foods reducing fat build-up in the body. Because of these properties, lemon juice is believed to reduce possible appearance of fatty lumps like lipoma through healthy elimination of toxins and excess fats in the body.

Another recommended alternative solution to treat lipoma and prevent its growth is flaxseed oil. Some health experts recommend regular intake of flaxseed oil because it is highly rich in omega-3 fatty acids. According to some studies, omega-3 fatty acids have properties that may effectively reduce or shrink fatty lumps under the skin and prevent growth of benign tumors.

If you think that you are prone to lipoma since one or two of your family members already have the condition, then healthy diet, proper exercise, and healthy lifestyle are definitely recommended. Since there are no known causes of lipomas yet, there are also no solid prevention measures to fight appearance and growth of lipoma.

The only solid preventive measure advised by health experts would be to eat the right foods to boost the immune system and avoid foods that would trigger the condition. Exercise is also highly recommended to healthily eliminate toxins and reduce fats, which can trigger growth of fatty lumps under the skin.

CHAPTER 6

# Symptoms of Lipoma

A part from the visible unsightly tumor growing slowly over a period of time, there are other symptoms of Lipoma. So look out for these symptoms and possible side effects, and then make an appointment with a doctor, if necessary.

## Early signs

Lipomas are asymptomatic, soft and mobile lumps under your skin. A Lipoma normally shows up as a soft lumpy growth, which is painless. It may be just one lump or a number of lumps together.

Many people disregard the presence of Lipomas, because they do not notice the slow growth over a long period of time. It is only when this growth begins to get ungainly that they notice and unsightly, fatty tumor at the back of their neck, on their shoulders, arms, legs or back. Some even have facial Lipomas.

A Lipoma is about the size of a small soft, fleshy marble anywhere between 1 to 3 centimeters in diameter. If left undisturbed, it may grow up to six centimeters, or even more. Its texture is rubbery and you are not going to feel any pain unless you squeeze it really hard.

## Classifying the Stages of Lipoma

It takes a long time for this benign tumor to grow. That is why it is normally disregarded by a number of people who overlook this slow and steady growth until the lumpy mass starts protruding from below the skin in a protuberant lump.

You are going to see Lipomas in just one lump or in a number of lumps together. They are going to be anywhere between 1 to 3 centimeters in diameter. They may even grow up to 10 centimeters in diameter. You need to get these Lipomas tested by a doctor as soon as possible so that he can prescribe the best treatment for your particular case.

## Common Features of Lipoma

Lipomas are painless. They grow very slowly and that is the reason why many people do not know that this tumor has been growing steadily over a given period of time on some part of their body. That is because Lipomas do not create discomfort until and unless they disfigure your body, – causing psychological and emotional discomfort – or start to press on your nerves.

# CHAPTER 7

# Diagnosis of lipoma

## Physical examination

Most skin experts like physicians and dermatologists just conduct a physical examination when determining a lipoma. They will feel the lumps and try to move it with their fingers to properly feel the growing lump of tissues under the skin. Physical examinations for diagnosing lipoma may also involve pinching or pressing of the lumps so medical professionals can determine the consistency of the tumor. Since lipomas are composed of fatty cells, they usually result in a dimpled appearance when being squeezed or pinched.

# Radiological Imaging

There are a number of state-of-the-art tests, which are going to help the doctor diagnose the presence of a lipoma in your colon, or somewhere else in your body.

An imaging or ultrasound test, especially in the form of a thorough and systematic CT or MRI scan is normally done by your doctor, if the lipoma is large, is deep-seated and has potential chances of being a liposarcoma.

> This is cancerous tissue and is definitely not a Lipoma, even though it looks like it. Lipomas are benign fatty deposits. A liposarcoma normally stays fixed in one place and does not move around like a Lipoma does. Also, it is painful and grows rapidly.

# Laboratory examination

For a proper diagnosis of a lipoma, the doctor is going to do a physical examination. After that he is going to take a bit of tissue for proper Lab examination. This is known as a biopsy. This is going to prove whether this is a benign lipoma or a possible cancerous growth known as liposarcoma. Liposarcoma diagnosis is usually confirmed after MRI, and Ultrasound scans.

### *Why should you get an immediate lipoma biopsy test done?*

Apart from getting to know about the nature of the tumor growth, – whether it is benign or not – your doctor will be able to decide whether a surgical removal is necessary or not. If the tumor mass is in an area where it has the potential to affect other organs, there is going to be immediate need to excise and remove that mass as soon as possible. If the lipoma does not affect your physical appearance or your internal system by affecting the organs or the nerves, surgical removal may not be necessary.

---

## Diagnosis Through Biopsy

If somehow the doctor is still in doubt about the real condition or cannot determine properly if the lump is indeed lipoma or can be other type of skin condition, then a lipoma biopsy may be recommended. Lipoma biopsy includes extraction of parts of the growing fatty cells for laboratory examination. Biopsy is done in order to accurately determine if the tumor under the skin is just a benign lump like lipoma or could be other serious conditions like cancer.

Biopsy is usually advised on order to be extra sure of the actual nature of the tumors growing under the skin. This skin examination is usually done by cutting through the skin, by getting tissue samples or it can also be done without incision by just extracting cell samples using a needle.

Once proper diagnosis is done and confirms the non-cancerous fatty lump as lipoma, patients can then decide to undergo either treatment or removal of the lipoma, or to leave it as it is. As mentioned above, lipomas are not cancerous and it will not also develop into malignant tumors. Lipomas also do not cause growth of other lumps in other parts of the body. If you have multiple lipomas, then that is another type of lipoma. Removal of lipoma may only be recommended if the lump becomes painful, infected, and cause problems to movements and proper functioning.

---

## Self-Assessment at Home

You can recognize a Lipoma on your own at home, when you see a soft lumpy growth under the surface of your skin. This growth is going to be on your arms, legs, shoulders, back, face or your chest region. A Lipoma has a spongy feel, when you press it. It does not cause you any sort of pain, because this is a benign tumor. Nevertheless, it is necessary that you go and see a doctor for a proper physical exam.

# Common Misdiagnosis for Lipoma

## Breast cancer

Some doctors may misdiagnose lipoma into a more serious condition like breast cancer due to the somewhat similar symptoms the two conditions share, which is the growing of lumps under the skin. Breast cancer can usually be detected when there is a lump within or just around the breast under the skin. These lumps are usually not easily detected because the lumps are too small so proper breast examination is needed in order to accurately diagnose and detect the condition.

## Lumps from Breast Fibroadenoma

Another common misdiagnosis for lipoma is breast fibroadenoma. This condition, just like lipoma, is also a non-malignant tumor and characterized by a breast lump. Just like the fatty lumps in lipoma, the breast lumps caused by breast fibroadenoma are also not tender and move easily when being pressed by the fingers.

# Lipoma Undiagnosed Conditions

Most people would get afraid when they notice or feel a lump just under the skin. Some women would think of breast cancer when they feel a lump just around the breast while some would think of skin cancer when there is lump growing just under the skin in other parts of the body. However, most of the skin diseases or conditions people suffer today are growing lumps between the skin and the muscle layers that are actually non-malignant or not cancerous.

# Why Lipomas Are Often Undiagnosed

Lipomas tend to be undiagnosed often basically because they grow really slow plus they can also be unfelt all throughout its growth especially for the lumps that grew in hidden or unnoticeable areas of the body like the back. People can sometimes only determine that they already have lipoma when they start to notice the lump or when the fatty tissues' size becomes noticeable.

Most lipoma is commonly diagnosed in men and women with middle age or sometimes during the elderly stage but the condition has actually been there for years. At the early stage of the condition, the lipomas or the fatty lumps can be really too small to notice. And if they do not inflict pain or discomfort or grow in parts of the body that are not commonly exposed, then there is great possibility that the lumps will continue to grow unnoticed for years.

Lipomas can even retain their size for years and grow really slowly making them hard to notice for years. Most lipomas that were diagnosed early are those lumps that grew near the nerves resulting to pain or those lumps that appeared in major airways of the body causing difficulty of breathing. Some diagnosed lipomas tend to also be found in sensitive areas of the body like the armpits and the thighs sometimes causing discomfort and difficulty in movement.

If the lipoma appeared in the face or the neck, then there is high possibility that this condition can be diagnosed during the early stage since most people would notice something different on their face or neck since this is a very commonly exposed part of the body.

Since lipomas are not cancerous tumors, some people who have this condition prefer not to have it treated or removed especially if the tumor does not cause pain or cause disturbance in the person's daily functioning and basic life. However, treatment may be required if the fatty lumps become infected or inflamed, or may start to release smelly discharge.

# CHAPTER 8

# Exploring Specific Causes

## Prevalence and Common Risk Factors

### Age

Apart from the risk of lipoma developing in those people who already are vulnerable to this condition through genetic inheritance, age also plays an important role in the possible appearance of this benign, soft, and spongy growth.

> Lipomas occur very rarely in children and babies, unless they are genetically prone to this condition. Women in the 30 – 48 age groups may suffer from solitary lipomas .Colon Lipomas may appear in women aged from 50 to 60. Men in the age group of 30 to 50 may develop lipomatosis – multiple lipomas.

As long as the lipoma is not painful, does not hinder your daily activities and is not in a sensitive internal region which may possibly affect any other organ, ask your doctors to keep monitoring it. He may then recommend surgical removal. Alternatively, he may suggest liposuction or steroid treatments to reduce its size, shape and look.

Even though the causes of Lipoma are unknown, there are some risk factors and diseases that are known to increase the chances of developing a Lipoma.

Apart from age, there are also some other factors which are going to influence the possibility of the emergence of a lipoma condition in a patient. Genetic inheritance can cause Gardner syndrome, familial multiple lipomatosis, and adiposis Dolorosa. Middle Age is also another factor which can give rise to the possibility of a Lipoma growth.

## Health Conditions

Your health is one of the most important factors, influencing the possibility of a lipoma growth in your body. People following a healthy lifestyle with plenty of exercise and eating nutritious and regular meals are going to be less prone to any sort of hormonal or biophysiological imbalances in their bodies. Overweight middle-aged adults – male or female – are more prone to lipomas. These growths normally occur in regions, where one is genetically programmed to have a natural fatty buildup. These areas include the shoulders, back, chest, waist, arms and thigh regions. In fact, lipomas can occur anywhere in your body where there is a layer of excess fat.

Here are some suggestions which are going to come in useful, when you are looking for the best and healthy diet to prevent, reduce or cure a Lipoma growth. Artificial sweeteners are out, because they have saccharin and aspartame. High fructose corn syrup is also definitely not good for your health. Include chemically refined sugar, foods with high chemical preservative percentage, etc. foodstuffs which have been preserved with nitrates and nitrites, including meat products should be avoided.

Increase your intake of natural and organic foods, and try out homeopathic and herbal remedies. They are not proven scientifically, but they are going to keep you healthy. Also, you can experiment with alternative medicine remedies, especially holistic diets and health care routines which cure the problem from the root onwards. This is going to be a time taking procedure, but it is going to be beneficial to you in the long run.

This natural and healthy diet is going to boost up your metabolism, detoxify your body, as well as in your and endocrine system, which may be responsible for the natural imbalance in your body, thus causing lipomas. If your health has started to deteriorate due to alcohol and tobacco abuse over a long period of time, you may find a biochemical imbalance in your natural system. Such a situation is conducive to lipoma growths.

# CHAPTER 9

# Lipoma Treatment

## Is There a Cure?

## Treatment Options

Patients with this condition can choose from various types of treatments available with removal through surgery as the most common option. Surgical removal of lipomas usually involves minor operation done in outpatient clinics and offices unless the lipoma is hard to reach and require the actual surgical procedure done in hospitals.

Aside from surgery, steroid injections are also available although this option only removes the lumps but does not completely treat the tumor. Liposuction is another common treatment recommended by dermatologists to remove lipomas. If you want to avoid invasive procedures, then there is also an alternative treatment known as the lipomassage therapy.

# Conventional Treatment Methods to remove Lipoma

Nowadays, there are a lot of available treatments or procedures for the removal of lipomas. Most patients who want to undergo the removal procedure prefer to have the benign tumors removed because the fatty lumps became painful and tender to the touch. Removal or treatment may also be necessary if the lipomas became inflamed or infected.

## Reasons For Undergoing Excision Of Lipoma

### *Cosmetic reasons:*

When the lipomas grow in obvious areas like the face and neck, it becomes insightful and embarrassing. And if they becomes inflamed, infected, and painful causing discomfort to the person. When the lipoma starts to release foul-smelling discharge, treatment may become necessary.

## *Movement Impairment:*

When the lipoma is situated in the sensitive area of the body causing pain or restriction to the movements like near the nerves, the vital organs, or the spine, and when the lipoma becomes too large, noticeable, and unsightly, when the lipoma starts to restrict movements or affect the function of the person due to its size and discomfort. Then treatment would be recommended.

## *Infection:*

Lipomas may also need to be surgically removed if it starts to show discharges that are quite foul smelling which can lead to embarrassment and may require covering and treatment.

## Surgical removal

Surgical removal of Lipomas are recommended by your doctor only if they find that the growth of the Lipoma may possibly be rise to a condition known as adiposis dolorosa, which is quite painful. Also, if they find the Lipoma changing its character or turning into possibly cancerous tissue, doctors are going to remove this fat fleshy growth surgically.

A small incision is going to be made in the affected area and the doctor is going to remove the tumor as far as possible. Some of these tumors are deep-seated and cannot be removed completely. Others may be in areas where it is difficult to reach them, without affecting other internal organs. In such cases, doctors remove the Lipoma portions to which they have easy access and leave the other dangerously situated portions of the Lipoma alone.

The incision is going to be sutured and bandaged. Doctors try their best to prevent scarring. During this surgical removal procedure, you may either be given a local anesthesia,- as in cases of small tumors – or a general anesthesia depending on the seriousness of the procedure and the size of the tumor.

You will need to stay on in the hospital for some days after the operation is done, if the Lipoma is large. It is a straightforward procedure, and normally does not give rise to any sort of side effects, if it is done proper-

ly and all the Lipoma tissue has been removed me-
thodically and systematically.

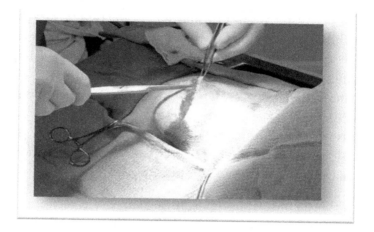

Remember that they can be potential complications in
some cases following lipoma surgery and that is the
reason why many people are going in for nonsurgical
procedures like liposuction and steroid injections.
These complications include – surgical infection, clot
formation, injury to the nerves because of permanent
anesthesia, injury to the nearby muscles and blood
vessels, scarring, and even possible permanent de-
formity in an organ, if the lesion is really large.

All this is definitely going to be prevented if you have
an experienced surgeon removing the tumor.

## Excision of Lipoma In Hospitals

Although not commonly done, some surgeons may also perform excision of lipomas in hospital's surgical facilities. These kinds of major surgical procedures for the removal of lipoma are done for lipomas are that situated in difficult areas of the body or parts that are quite harder to reach where basic excision of lipomas is not possible anymore. These difficult locations can be near a joint, an artery, the spine, near the nerve, or close to vital organ where precise and complex removal is necessary to avoid complications.

For these kinds of lipomas, major surgery removal will be needed and needs to be done in the hospitals or in inpatient surgery facilities. Major operations for the removal of lipoma may also require general anesthesia to make the patients unconscious during the procedure. For lipomas located near sensitive and difficult areas like in vital organs, careful and precise removal of lipoma without affecting surrounding tissues is definitely important to avoid complications.

Before the excision of lipoma, surgeons or medical professionals that will be performing the procedure usually advise the patients to relax for a few days before the day of procedure so the body is prepared for the surgery. Patients who are scheduled to undergo the excision of lipoma are also advised to avoid lifting heavy objects or standing for long hours few days before the procedure. Aside from excision of lipoma, another common option preferred by patients to remove lipoma is liposuction.

## Steroid injections

Steroid injections are nonsurgical methods in which you can get a Lipoma removed. This is going to cause the shrinkage of the Lipoma growth, but it also means that you have to take these injections over a long period of time. Also, this does not remove the Lipoma growth completely. Remember; get your steroid injections done by an experienced doctor.

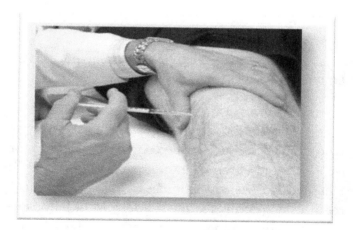

## Liposuction

If you want to avoid invasive procedures like surgeries and the possible scar, you can also opt for liposuction.

However, just like steroid injections, liposuction can only reduce the appearance of the lump or shrink the bump but does not completely remove the tumors.

## Laser Treatment

Laser treatment for lipoma is one of the latest treatments available for the removal of lipomas. Unlike surgeries, laser treatments use heat to burn, shrink the lumps beneath the skin, and leave minimal to no scar to the skin. However, laser treatments for the removal of lipoma may only be applicable for small size lipomas.

## Lipomassage Therapy

Lipomassage is also one of the latest solutions for lipoma. This option is perfect for people with lipomas who do not want to undergo invasive surgeries or injections, and prefer alternative options like lipomassage. However, lipomassage therapies usually require long-term treatment and just like liposuction and injections, lipomassage may only be effective in reducing the size of the lumps but does not effectively remove the tumors.

## Preparing for an appointment

Preparing for an appointment with your doctor about the possibility of a lipoma condition should never be a traumatic experience. Your doctor is experienced and knowledgeable. He is good to give you the best advice, and that is why he is going to make a proper diagnosis. After that, it is possible that he is going to recommend you to a good dermatologist for possible surgical removal of the Lipoma

You want to get some questions ready before you go and see your doctor –Symptoms – write down any symptoms, including nausea, headaches, fever, possible gastrointestinal bleeding, fatigue, etc. They may or may not be related to your condition, but they are going to give your doctor a good idea of what is wrong with you. Of course he can visibly see the lipoma. He may recommend a biopsy or diagnostic imaging CT or MRI scan which is going to be done by testing your tissue sample. It is wise to write down all the symptoms. Please do not exaggerate any hide symptoms.

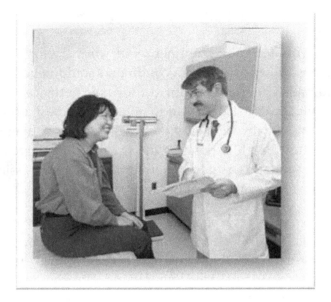

Make a list of all the drugs that you are taking. Some drugs may cause side effects, which may have aggravated the lipoma growth. Also include any supplements, medications and vitamins that you are taking.

You may want to ask your doctor some questions about the lipoma, whether it is a potentially life threatening condition [no, it is not...] and whether it is cancerous tissue. [Again, no it is not...] Write these questions down.

You may also want to ask him about the reasons for this growth, whether your lifestyle has anything to do with it [increased alcohol consumption may affect lipoma growth], whether it is genetically inherited and your children may also carry the lipoma gene, removal and treatment of the lipoma and the risk factors. The doctor is going to give you all the information required about the lipoma, its growth, treatment and removal and necessary tests needed to confirm this benign tumor as a lipoma.

## Other symptoms which may or may not be related to lipoma

Here are some other symptoms which may or may not be related to lipoma, and may concern your general state of health and mind. Look out for the symptoms and do tell your doctor about them-

Depression,

Inability to concentrate,

Change in regular bowel movements,

Headaches,

Absentmindedness,

Change in body temperature,

Numbness in body extremities,

State of mental confusion,

Sensitive skin, which bruises easily.

These are just some common symptoms which you would like to note down. Your doctor is going to take them into account too, when he is diagnosing a possible lipoma condition.

Your doctor is going to ask you a number of questions which include –

When did you see this lump?

Is it painful?

How long since it has been growing?

Do you have a history of such growths in your family?

Have you ever suffered from lipomas before?

What are the medicines you are taking for other possible ailments?

These are just some of the questions which the doctor would like to know before he recommends a lab test or an imaging test. After that, he is going to diagnose the condition and recommend the best possible treatment for you. So book an appointment with your doctor right now and talk to him about that lipoma growth on your body.

## Alternative Solutions For Lipoma

Although there are no studies that would prove the efficacy of alternative solutions, some patients have provided positive feedback about alternative medicines and treatments developed for the treatment of lipoma. One popular alternative option available today is lipomassage wherein the lumps or tumors are prevented from growing through massage therapies.

Application of natural topical concoctions and extracts are also recommended by some patients who have lipomas and experienced reduced pain through the application of these topical products like turmeric and olive oil, and castor oil. To reduce the size of lipomas and prevent them from growing, some patients and health experts recommend patients to regularly apply castor oil several times a day.

The combination of olive oil and paste of turmeric is also recommended by some herbal experts because of its abilities to soften and reduce lumps in the skin. Some health experts would also recommend proper diet and intake of specific foods that are theorized to effectively reduce size of lipomas and prevent growth like lemon juice, flaxseed oil, and avoidance of fatty foods.

# CHAPTER 10

# Non-Surgical and Alternative Methods

There are some Lipoma treatments, including natural remedies which lack scientific evidence. In fact, what works for one person may not work for other, because both of them have different bio-physiological compositions However, natural remedies like turmeric, Sage, vitamins D and E in fresh and organically grown fruit and vegetables, pure soda bicarbonate, chickweed, almond seeds [limited to just one or two, because they contain harmful natural ingredients] are just some of the natural remedies which are being recommended on the Internet as cures, aids and treatment for lipomas.

There are plenty of other homeopathic and Ayurvedic natural remedies which are being used in India down the ages to treat tumors and other skin conditions. But because they do not have scientific evidence, they are not considered as conventional treatment methods in the West.

Here are treatments which lack scientific evidence, but it has excellent logical explanations as to its efficacy – detoxification of your body. Get rid of the toxin buildup in your body and you are going to find a significant positive effect on your health

## Detoxification Recipes

Here are some detoxification recipes which are very common in the East, they keep the system healthy. Fresh Lemon juice on an empty stomach taken first thing every morning is one of the best ways in which you can detoxify your body. It also prevents constipation. Drink plenty of fresh fruit juice whenever you can, instead of coffee or alcohol. Not only does this keep your system healthy, but it detoxifies your body wonderfully well.

Herbs like Sage and spices like turmeric should be added to your food. Not only do they detoxify your body, but they also prevent toxin buildup over a given period of time. Add lot of natural vitamins brought to you naturally in fruit and vegetables to your daily diet. Never stint on any important food group through dieting. Dieting or missing out on meals is one of the most harmful ways in which you can upset your body's natural bio-physiological system and rhythm.

A good detoxifying cleansing method will never recommend you to eat just one particular group of food items over a given period of time. Exercising is going to get rid of the fat content in your body. Supported with a proper and healthy diet, with all the essential vitamins, nutrients and minerals required to keep your body healthy, you may find yourself losing body fat. This fat has given way to muscles. It also means that the fatty tumor has been reduced because the liver needs those fat cells to produce energy, which was burned up during an exercise routine.

## Helpful Natural Products

Here is a list of helpful natural products, including spices and herbs on which doctors are researching, they believe them to be helpful in curing Lipoma, and they are still lack of sufficient scientific evidence to prove the effectiveness of these natural products.

Aloe

Arginine

Beta-carotene

Black cohosh

Chocolate-dark unsweetened black, chocolate, also known as bitter chocolate is being researched as a good product to help reduce lipomas.

Chondroitin sulfate

Coca

Coenzyme Q10

Cranberry

Creatine

DHEA.

Dong quai

Echinacea

Ephedra

Evening primrose oil

Flaxseed and flaxseed oil

Folate

Ginkgo

Glucosamine

Honey

Lactobacillus acidophilus

Lycopene

Melatonin

Milk thistle

Niacin

Omega-3 fatty acids, fish oil, alpha-linolenic acid – any fish, which is rich in omega-3, including salmon, oysters, lobsters, tuna, sardines, mackerel are extremely good for your heart, as well as for your health. Make them an important and regular part of your diet.

Red yeast rice

SAMe

Saw palmetto

Soy

St. John's wort

Tea tree oil

Thiamin

Vitamin A

Vitamin B12

Vitamin B6

Vitamin C

Vitamin D

Vitamin E

Whey protein

Zinc

## Acupuncture In Lipoma Treatment

Acupuncture is also an alternative medicine form, which even though not scientifically proven is considered to be helpful in relieving some Lipoma symptoms. Acupuncture goes deep into the art of natural body balance. Balancing a disturbed system by treating the disturbed regions with the help of little needles is considered to be a good way to restore health.

Acupuncture has been in existence for thousands of years and experienced acupuncture masters have been treating Lipoma down the centuries in China. So it would not do you any harm to try out this alternative medicine science to cure your body's natural imbalance of the life force and set it in harmony again.

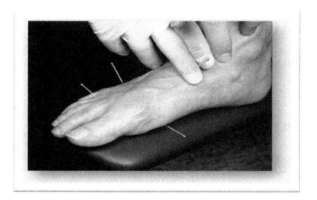

# Natural and Home Remedies

Natural and home remedies for effective and proper Lipoma treatment have been in existence for millenniums. But they are time consuming and that is the reason why many impatient people do not bother about trying to get rid of this ill from the roots, as is done through alternative medicine mediums.

## Ayurveda

Here are some recommendations which you may try out. Ayurveda, also known as Ayurvadic medicine is a system of traditional medicine which has been in existence for 3000 years. Turmeric is one of the spices which is very popular in Eastern cuisine. It is only now that the West has found out that it has cancer preventing properties. Here is one treatment, which lacks scientific evidence as to efficacy, but is considered to be a really good and effective treatment.

## Turmeric, Milk and Honey

A paste of turmeric, milk and honey is applied to the Lipoma directly and regularly in order to produce a noticeable reduction in that fatty mass over a given period of time.

Turmeric is capable of staining your clothes so beware

When Eastern herbalists and beauticians were asked about the efficacy of this procedure, they said that turmeric has long been known as a skin beautifying agent. Honey is a natural antiseptic and moisturizer. The skin is massaged slowly after the application of this herbal paste. Logic says that the breaking up of the fat cells during the massage is largely responsible for the reduction of this tumor. The reason is simple and rational.

## Dandelion and Chickweed Powder

You may want to steep two teaspoons each of dandelion and chickweed powder in hot boiling water. This tea is an effective way in which you can reduce the size of Lipomas.

## Thujaoccidentalis

Thujaoccidentalis is a plant which grows very prominently in India. Its extract is commonly used for treating skin problems in Indian Ayurvedic medicine. Take five drops of Thuja Extract, add some water to it, and massage it into your Lipoma three times a day. You are going to see definite visible effects within a couple of months.

Natural remedies normally take a long time to show visible effects, because they are treating the problem externally, instead of going to the root of the matter. So be patient and try these remedies out.

## 5 Good Detoxifying /Body Cleansing Foods

Did you know that the ancients in Asia went through a rigorous detoxifying and body cleansing ritual at periodic intervals every year? This is when they ate special foods to allow the body to get rid of all the accumulated toxins. This ritual ceremony of getting rid of all the toxins through fasting and eating special detoxifying foods is still followed by a large multitude of people in India today. This fasting period continues for 10 days and takes place twice a year.

Why it is necessary for the body to get rid of toxins periodically? Just imagine that you have been eating lots of proteins throughout a given period of time. It is hard for your digestive system to digest proteins.

Your digestive system has digested just a portion of the meat. Also, there are some toxic wastes which still remain in your body even after a protein-based meal has been digested and eliminated. That is why you may find yourself feeling sluggish and lethargic even 24 to 48 hours after a heavy meat-based meal. That is because a portion of the protein still stays in your system in the shape of toxins.

These are the toxins which need to be removed regularly through detoxification. Otherwise, they are going to have a detrimental effect on the chemical and physiological systems of your body. That long accumulating affect is also going to affect your physical and mental well-being in the long run.

Shakespeare could not have said it better. In Twelfth night, Act I, scene 3, Sir Andrew Aguecheek says," but I am a keen eater of beef, and I believe that does serious harm to my wits". That is the reason why the wise ancients of the East and West preferred a fruit and vegetable diet over a meat diet, millenniums ago. That meant that they did not need to detoxify their bodies ever so often.

So what are the best detoxifying/body cleansing foods available in nature today?

## Apples

Let us start with one of the best detoxifying foods available to us – the Apple. An apple a day keeps the doctor away. It also keeps the dentist away because the malic acid in the apple is supposed to keep your teeth healthy and strong. You may notice young children crunching apples regularly to have glowing complexions, healthier white teeth and sturdy little bodies. That is because their bodies are being regularly detoxified due to a regular intake of organic apples.

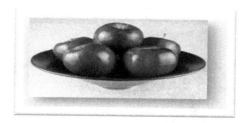

Please look for organic detoxifying food items to prevent more toxic pesticide accumulation in your body.

## Yoghurt and buttermilk.

Have you tried adding large portions of yogurt to your daily diet? People in the East have made sure that yogurt and buttermilk are an integral part of their normal day- to- day meals. Buttermilk is a tasty, healthy, rejuvenating and appetizing drink. Yogurt has a number of probiotic bacteria which help in digestion and cleansing the body's physiological systems.

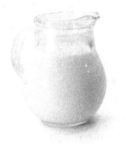 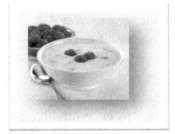

## Leafy Green

Greens are always on the top of one's detoxifying lists, but Popeye had the best idea. A regular dose of lots and lots of spinach kept him healthy and strong. Spinach is one of the best detoxifying foods available to you today. Other leafy greens in the spinach family and greens like alfalfa, wheatgrass have plenty of chlorophyll. Chlorophyll can get rid of all the accumulated metals and toxins present in your body. Well-cooked spicy spinach is nutritious as well as delicious, so you cannot get away with an excuse that spinach is not tasty at all. So bring on the Greens.

## Citrus fruits

Citrus fruits, especially oranges and limes are excellent detoxers. Here is a time-tested recipe for a lemon squash drink, which is drunk in copious amounts all through the summer by people in the East. It is simply called lemon water! Try it out right now and prevent your body from getting dehydrated. Also, it is perfect for detoxifying your body.

Squeeze out the juice of four juicy lemons. Put this juice in 8 cups of water. You may add the zest of the lemons to this water too, if you like your lime juice slightly more sour. Allow this water to boil for about four minutes, remove, strain the lemon juice and add honey to taste. Top with lots of ice cubes and enjoy. Some people also enjoy lemon slices in this lemon water. You may also try it with salt and pepper instead of honey.

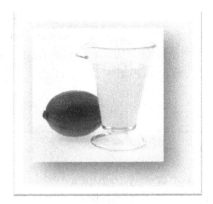

Citrus fruits are excellent body cleansing agents. They are also good sources of vitamin C, preventing scurvy and colds. They are excellent reasons for your bright eyes, glowing complexion, healthy immunity system and good teeth. So remember to add lots of citrus fruit in your daily diet.

Herbs like ginger and garlic are good body cleansing agents. Garlic is a mild antiseptic. A paste of onions, ginger and garlic may not smell so appealing to Western tastes. But it is an integral and very healthy part of Eastern and Middle Eastern cuisine, not only for its flavorsome tang, but also for its detoxifying qualities. This paste is also known as masala.

Here we come to another body cleansing spice, which is an important part of healthy cuisine – turmeric.

## Turmeric

Turmeric has long been known as a spice which prevents cancer, which adds flavor to your ginger, garlic and onion masala and which detoxifies your body. The ubiquitous curry powder found in American markets has lots of turmeric added in it, and which is being marketed as authentic, original Asian curry masala. However, here is the original Eastern curry powder recipe which consists of 8 tablespoons of cumin seed powder, 2 tablespoons each of ginger and onion powder, 3 tablespoons of turmeric, chili powder, according to your tastes and how spicy you want the curry powder to be and 6 tablespoons of coriander powder.

Good cooks normally fry these powders (except turmeric) on a griddle beforehand to "set"the aroma and flavor. Grind them together and put them in a glass airproof jar to preserve their aromatic properties for a longer period of time. Use half a teaspoon of this curry powder to add zing to your food, knowing that you are eating healthy and detoxifying spices.

## Bean sprouts

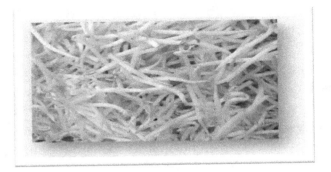

Bean sprouts, especially mung bean sprouts are very effective detoxifying food items. Place them in a bowl on your table, with a little bit of salt, pepper, cayenne pepper and lemon juice mixed in the beams topped up with some olive oil. Remember to grab a handful upon which to choose whenever you pass the table. Try using this snack as the filler between meals instead of potato chips and other junk food.

You can always add more delicious detoxifying food items like nuts and seeds – walnuts, sultanas, raisins, sunflower seeds, peanuts and other seeds – to the bean sprouts to make this salad more appetizing.

So now that you know all about the most effective body cleansing and detoxifying food items available in nature today, is not it time that you start to detoxify your body with these healthy and delicious foods?

# CHAPTER 11

# Physical Exercise Approach to Lipoma removal

Some experts argued the capability of exercises in reducing or removing lipomas. That is on the premise that lipomas are caused by chemical imbalances or are inherited. However, there are some evidence that have proven that proper diet and exercising help to increase your metabolism and encourage your liver and gallbladder to burn the fat cells present in your body, thereby helping to reduce fatty lumps. Since lipomas are mainly fatty lumps, reducing body fat may lead to reduction in the size of the lipomas.

It is sensible to reduce your body fat, especially around your waist, back, shoulders and chest region as a matter of a natural and practical good health routine. A proper exercise routine is thus going to tone up your body. Exercising means that your body's metabolism rate has increased, and your liver is burning up more fat cells. So here are some tips and exercises that are not only going to reduce your body fat, but will also shrink Lipoma lumps in the long run. It is almost impossible to drop 2 sizes overnight. It took about 3 to 5 months, on average to put on those inches slowly and steadily.

## Factors Leading To Overweight

Did you change your diet? Have you started eating some food items, which were full of calories and fat content? Did you reduce on your carbohydrate and protein intake? Or did you start skipping your meals in order to lose stomach fat? These are just some of the factors which are going to influence the presence of fat, around your waist region. So, make a list of the food and the drinks that you have been taking this past week. Have you increased your beer intake? This is going to give you an estimation of the calories which you are consuming on a daily basis. If they are more than what your body needs, it is going to show up as cellulite deposits around your stomach, thighs and hips.

Now you know all about the amount of calories that you have been taking steadily through these months, you need to reduce all those foods which have been providing you with these undesirable energy laden calories. You will have to reduce your calorie intake from anywhere between 700 to 800 cal per day, in order to get your metabolism working properly. Also, once this calorie reduction has been done, your body is going to start burning up the cellulite cells, in order to provide the body with the necessary energy.

Support your metabolism's cell burning activities by exercising your muscles. When you do physical work, the muscles demand energy from the body. The calories are thus burned in a very natural manner. Try out an exercise session for a week, starting with walking a couple of miles per day, and then slowly and steadily increasing the distance and time. You are going to be surprised to see how your legs have lost weight, and yes, your stomach also seems to have lost some weight. This is visible and is going to be the best incentive for you to stay with this brisk exercise routine.

Any sort of energy reduction or deficit in your body means a slow and steady loss of stomach fat. Remember that this needs to be done consistently, for it to show visible and effective results. It is of no use tiring yourself out today and then losing all enthusiasm for continuing that same activity tomorrow, because all your muscles are protesting and groaning.

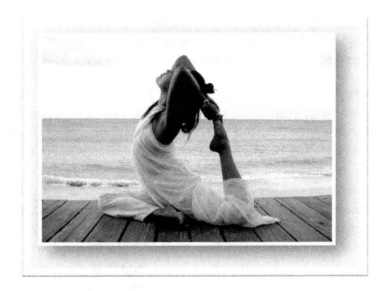

You may also want to try out yoga and exercises to get rid of the fat and build up the muscles.

A well-toned body with minimal fat content is not conducive to a Lipoma buildup. Also, you may want to add more proteins, carbohydrates and fresh fruits and vegetables to your diet. These essential natural nutrients are good to improve your general health and tone up your bio- physiological system.

Lipomas are made up of fatty cells, and that is why you need to have a good metabolism, which can break down the fat in a natural manner. Look at the good ways in which you can increase your metabolic rate – like exercise – and see the improvement in your general health.

# Dieting and Lipoma

There is no enough scientific evidence for this supposition, but some food experts believe that diet can have a positive or negative effect on Lipomas. In fact, fresh fruit and fresh vegetables, omega-3 rich fish, Sage and other natural herbs, normally used in alternative medical treatments like Ayurveda were found to have to have a positive effect on Lipomas. The basis of this positive result is straightforward. Detoxify your body and continue with a healthy diet supported by proper exercise. This is going to heal your possibly disturbed biochemistry. This is thus naturally going to have a positive effect on a Lipoma growth.

People are trying out alternative methods like apricot juice and grape juice to get rid of Lipomas. There is no scientific basis for the success of such a natural remedies, but it is a well-known fact that these are good, anti-toxic agents. Also, you will need to drink fresh fruit juices and grape juice for a number of months to see any sort of possible diminishing of the Lipoma. Your body is being detoxified by your change in the diet, it is possible that toxin buildup and Lipoma buildup are intricately connected.

If fat loss with a change in the diet is your immediate priority, and you are looking for ways and means in which you can reduce body fat, well, here are some guaranteed effective fat loss tips, which bring positive results. This is going to have an effect on your Lipoma because after all this fatty mass is a collection of fatty cells and when you are looking for ways and means to get rid of these fatty cells through exercise and proper diet, there you are, there is going to be a visible reduction in your Lipoma's size and state.

Firstly, stop looking for magic and miraculous pills, potions and cures, which promise you a fat loss overnight. You cannot achieve fat loss through topical treatments or ingesting miraculous herbs and pills. It is a bio-physiological process. Any sort of weight loss overnight or within a couple of days is not considered to be healthy. It may mean that your body is suffering from some serious pathology, and rapid short term weight loss can be its danger signal.

It may also means that you are possibly starving in order to lose some weight. That is when your body goes into emergency action mode. It knows that it is not going to get any nutritive food supply in the next couple of days. It then starts storing up fat cells, which can then be converted into energy whenever required by the body. This fat deposit can be considered as your body's emergency store.

So you need to go about the fat loss procedure in a steady and systematic manner. Eat four small meals a day with plenty of proteins and carbs. Get your body metabolism to start working, instead of staying sluggish because it has nothing to do. This is going to be done by supporting your nutritive diet with at least half an hour of physical exercise every day. Not only does this get rid of all the toxins in the body, but it gets all your body muscles working. It is not mandatory that you go to a gym and work out on aerobic routines. Try walking, swimming, dancing, working in the garden in the sun, any activity which gets your muscles moving. Do not wear your body out in a burst of enthusiasm to lose weight rapidly.

What I am saying is do not go for drastic weight loss measures. Those hard dieting programs used by some celebrities and recommended by some "so called" weight loss experts online, may be harmful. They may destroy natural biochemical and bio-physiological balance; due to intense starvation. It has also not got the necessary ingredients and nutrients which are necessary to keep the body functioning in a healthy manner.

Go in for small steps in your weight loss program. A couple of pounds lost during the week is good. It means your body is getting used to the fact that weight loss and fat loss is being done in a proper and systematic manner.

So a little bit of perseverance and you are going to find visible and successful fat loss results all over your body. Your stomach, however, is going to take anywhere between six months to a year to look trim, but that is only going to be done if you have been eating properly and exercising consistently. Naturally, this means that you are going to see a significant physical improvement and visible difference in the size of Lipoma too.

# CHAPTER 12

# Managing Lipoma: Helpful Tips

## Living with a Person with Lipoma

Lipomas are not life-threatening. Nevertheless, these ugly looking growths are quite enough to cause young people who are very conscious about their appearance a lot of concern that can influence the family environment and atmosphere. That is because these young people may suffer from a low self-esteem and low self-confidence.

So if you have a family member who is suffering from Lipoma, you need to show them love and reassure. Also, you may help them try out natural remedies like massaging that area with warm almond oil or wheat germ oil at least once a day. This is going to have a long-term positive effect on the lipoma, because the fatty cells are going to break up in that area.

# Aids for People with Lipoma

There are no hundred percent successful over the counter aids for Lipoma reduction. On the other hand, there are many sites on the Internet, which promise to get rid of your Lipoma through herbal supplements and remedies. Your doctor is going to diagnosis a lipoma condition with the help of a CT or MRI scan supported by endoscopy or a tissue biopsy, if necessary. As this is not a cancerous tumor, it is going to get worrisome only when it begins to start paining, starts pressing on nerves or begins to grow, thus causing discomfort.

Excising the tumor in a surgical operation when recommended is a good way in which you can get rid of it. But this is when it is easily accessible and superficial. Herbal vitamins and supplements are useful to reduce the tumors. Some of these herbal extracts include ingredients like chickweed, Sage and lemon juice. Thujaofficianalis extract as a topical cream along with turmeric is a good way with which you can reduce the size of a Lipoma.

Chickweed tincture is normally taken as a teaspoon of chickweed powder in boiling water, three times a day. The Chinese use a paste made of chickweed directly upon the Lipoma, massaging that area and allowing the herb to get assimilated into the skin. Chickweed. Dried chickweed is found at herbalists shops.

I discovered that the increase of bitter foods in my daily diet caused my lipomas to shrink significantly. This is because these foods are good to break up the fat cells in your body by increasing its metabolic rate. The liver and gallbladder, thus gets toned up when you eat foods like gentian, yarrow, rue, bitter gourd, citrus peel, dandelions, golden seal, wormwood, and even dark chocolate!

Lemon juice and fresh orange juice is definitely the best way in which you can detoxify your body. Remember to chew the lemon and orange peel, afterwards. Apart from being good detox foods, they are also good to get rid of any harmful parasites in your digestive system.

Topical aids like creams containing cider vinegar are supposedly effective in controlling Lipoma in its early stages. You may also want to drink a teaspoon of natural cider vinegar in a glass of water a couple of times a day in order to clear your system and prevent Lipoma growths.

# CHAPTER 13

# Concluding Remarks

## A More Serious Problem

We have established that Lipomas are not dangerous or are benign tumors that are made up of fatty cells. But serious cases of lipomas could lead to bleeding in gastrointestinal tract, ulceration and as well as blockage in the areas of the body such as the throat. Lipomas are really needed to be removed if the person feels discomfort and pain. Complications such as inflamed and infected lipomas may also arise, characterized by a foul smelling discharged.

The complications of lipomas may threaten the health of a person, therefore, it is a must to surgically remove them. There is no known treatment or method in preventing the growth of lipomas. When lipomas grow excessively it may result to the decrease in the mobility of the person which in turn decrease the person's ability to function.

## Complications Due To Lipoma

The complication that may occur when an individual has a lipoma or lipomas depends on the location of the lump or tumor. Complication from a lipoma may only occur if it affects the surrounding tissue or organs of our body. Lipomas are not considered to be a serious medical problem. Lipomas can only become a problem if they grow excessively on some rare cases and press on the nerves on that area. The blockage or a pressured nerve is the one that produces pain and discomfort to a person with lipoma.

The large and painful lipomas must be dealt with accordingly in order to prevent more serious health issues that may arrived from such medical condition. You can cure lipoma by following the treatment plan provided by your health care provider or you can opt for a surgical removal of the tumor in order guarantee the immediate removal of pain and discomfort.

## Treating Lipoma To Avoid Complications

Most of the cases of lipomas do not necessarily require an immediate surgical operation or even a simple operation. Lipomas are generally harmless and only needs to be dealt with when they grow rapidly and causes pain, discomfort and stress to an individual. A cosmetic surgeon or a general surgeon can perform the said surgical operation for removing the lipomas. If your physician, doctor or health care provider diagnosed that the lump under your skin is not cancerous or benign, then the health care provider will come up with the best possible treatment in order to regain the lead. Some of the processes involve in removing lipomas include liposuction, steroid injections (shrinks the lipomas), and surgical procedures or incisions in order to remove the lipomas.

---

## Lipoma and Self Esteem

Unsightly Lipomas especially when they are on your face or on visible parts of your body can have an adverse effect on your self-esteem. If that is the case, you need to ask your doctor for the best remedy that he is going to suggest to you to get rid of this Lipoma. Remember that self-confidence is basically a matter of autosuggestion. Some people can auto suggests themselves into neurotic cases, just because they are very conscious about their appearance or they do not have a feeling of self-respect or self-esteem.

So if you think that an unsightly Lipoma is affecting the quality of your life and having a drastic effect on your mental health, contact your doctor immediately. You can opt for the treatment methods in which the Lipoma can be removed without leaving any scar. This can either be a cosmetic procedure through steroid injections, or it can be surgical removal.

Here is some more information about self-esteem. Some people are so conscious about themselves that they spend thousands of dollars getting themselves cosmetically enhanced in order to look more youthful and beautiful. If you think that getting that Lipoma removed – or any other surgical procedure may make you feel more happy, content and well satisfied with your life, make you feel more positive, make you feel more secure in yourself, well, then go for it.

---

# Chronic Inflammation in the Body

## *Lipoma and HIV*

Here are some of the scientific studies which have been done by eHealthMe about the statistics of the prevalence for lipoma development in HIV-infected people. 37,390 people were studied by the FDA for this report.

0.3 percent of these 37,390 people suffering from HIV infection have lipoma. On the other hand, lipoma is more common with people suffering from high blood pressure, rheumatoid arthritis, high blood cholesterol and which there is a disturbance in the body's fat metabolism. That means that there is going to be a complete absence of fat in your body, or perhaps you may find abnormal deposits of fat throughout your body.

This is a genetically inherited syndrome or can be caused due to HIV infection. The symptoms of this syndrome include absence of body fat, abnormally, thin arms and legs and dry skin.

Based on various studies, lipoma is definitely not related to HIV. Some researches study the possible connection of lipoma to HIV while some studies claim that lipoma can be a sign of HIV. However, there is no confirmed relationship between the two conditions yet. HIV or Human Immunodeficiency Virus is a lent virus that can lead to AIDS or the acquired immunodeficiency syndrome while lipoma is the slow-growing fatty acids underneath the skin with no confirmed causes yet, even HIV.

Although some people infected with HIV have lipomas, their percentage is only small and growth of the lumps cannot also be related directly to the virus. This is because some HIV-infected patients already had the lipomas even before they acquired the HIV. Lentivirus technology denied the claim that, HIV virus could be a possible cause of lipoma or the benign fatty lumps.

50 percent of the patients 30 to 39 age group and 50 percent of the patients in the 50 to 59 age group suffered from lipomas. 23.08 percent female patients suffered from lipomas compared to 76.92 percent male patients.

Pubic Lipomas or lipoma fat pad developments have been noted in HIV patients. These Pubic Lipomas are more common among obese women, and also in HIV infected persons. Medical associations are considering Pubic lipomas as a part of HIV-associated lipodystrophy syndrome. Lipodystrophy syndrome is a condition in which there is degeneration of the body tissues and it is now being considered as a possible sign of HIV infection.

## Lipoma And Medications For HIV

Some studies were also conducted in order to determine the relation of the specific drugs or medicines taken by HIV-infected patients to the development or risk of acquiring lipoma. Some HIV patients taking medicines like Zometa, Prednisone, Paxil, Fosamax, and Prilosec reported having lipoma but just like in other studies about the condition and its relation to HIV, the study also did not prove any solid relation between the drugs HIV patients were taking and the growth of lipomas.

This is because the number of cases reported are not sufficient to prove that the medications for HIV can trigger the development of lipoma, plus some patients may also already had the skin condition even before they started taking the medications for HIV.

As I mentioned earlier, lipoma is one of the many health problems present today that have no confirmed causes. Based on various studies, the most popular theory accepted by some medical experts on the cause of lipoma is genetics and hereditary. This is because lipoma has been found in family members and may have transferred from generation to generation.

Aside from hereditary and genetics, another possible cause of lipoma is injury. Some health and medical experts believe that injury or trauma in the skin can lead to the formation of fatty lumps in the skin or an injury in the skin can be a condition where the lumps may appear. Although it is a theorized possible cause of lipoma, there is also still no firm evidence that would prove that trauma or injury can be a direct cause of formation and development of lipoma.

## Lipoma Treatment and Insurance Coverage

Some people opt to go for surgical removal not because of the fear of complication from lipomas or the health issues it brings but because of the unsightly presence of the tumor. When lipomas are removed not because of the health threat, then some insurance companies in America, and Europe may not cover the cost of the surgery. Insurance companies will only cover the expenses of a lipoma surgery when the lipoma of a patient is proven to cause some complications such as restriction of movement, infection, pain and other more complications.

The removal of lipomas is usually done in the outpatient surgery center. The doctor applies local anesthesia around the area of the lipomas. The doctor then performs an incision on the skin in order to remove the tumor.

However, if the lipomas are deep under the skin or organ, general anesthesia is used on the patient and it is performed in a more suitable environment such as the operating room. Complications may also occur after the surgery but doctors will advise some ways on how to minimize or prevent possible complications.

# CHAPTER 14

# Lipoma FAQ

Lipoma affects millions of people around the world today. If you think that you have lipoma and want to know relevant facts about this condition, then here are answers to some of the most common questions asked about this skin disease.

### Is lipoma cancerous?

No. Lipoma is not a cancer. It is a benign tumor slowly growing underneath the skin.

### Can it develop into cancer?

No. Lipoma will not develop into cancer. The common complications of lipoma are infection, inflammation, and restricted movements.

### Is it contagious?

No. Lipomas are not contagious and do not also cause the appearance of lumps in other parts of the body.

## What are the causes of lipoma?

There are no known causes of lipoma yet but health experts believe that it can connected to genetics and heredity in humans.

## Why are some lipomas painful?

Sometimes, lipoma becomes painful because it grew near the nerves or blood vessels causing pinched nerves and inflammation.

## When to see a doctor?

Lipomas are rarely dangerous but if you notice some lumps on your skin or some areas where there were lumps became painful to touch, consult a doctor to have the lumps checked.

## What are the risk factors?

Lipomas are more common in men and women aging 40 to 60 years old but they can appear in people of all ages. People who have certain disorders can also be at higher risk of getting this condition such as people with Cowden syndrome, adiposis dolorosa, Gardner's syndrome, and Madelung disease.

## Do I need to undergo tests?

Most doctors and medical professionals can easily determine a lipoma from other more serious skin diseases like liposarcoma because of the consistency and specific distinct characteristics of benign lumps. Most doctors would only conduct thorough physical examination and get your medical records. However, if you want to be sure that the lumps are only lipoma then you can also undergo tests like biopsy or other imaging tests like CT scan and MRI.

### Are the lumps permanent?

Yes. Lipoma is a permanent condition.

### Can the lumps be removed permanently?

Yes. Lipomas can be removed through various treatments like laser therapy, liposuction, steroid injection, and excision surgery. One of the most common treatments to remove lipoma is surgical removal or more commonly known as excision of lipoma. Removal of lipomas usually require minor operations with local anesthesia only, since most lipomas are located in areas that are easy to reach and operate with like the neck, the back, the shoulder, arms and legs. However, for lipomas in difficult and complicated areas like near vital organs, major surgery may be required and must be performed in the hospital surgical facility.

### Can lipoma re-occur after removal?

Some lipomas return after removal but the possibility of relapse depends on the kind of treatment you have undergone. Surgical removal is the most effective solution to remove lipomas and has been reported to have the least reoccurrence among other treatments after the removal.

### What are the ways to prevent lipoma?

Since there are no confirmed causes yet of lipoma, there are also no known prevention measures to fight the development of this condition.

### Is Lipoma Contagious?

Lipomas are not cancerous. They are really harmless and also not contagious. Some medical experts believe that lipomas can be hereditary. Lipomas can be present in your body for so many years unnoticed until you can really notice the bulge. This type of medical condition can grow in the different part of your body at the same time but it does not necessary mean that it is contagious.

Having a lipoma is not a serious health threat since it is a benign or non-cancerous tumor and the condition is also not a threat to other people who came in contact with the person with lipomas. According to studies, one lipoma does not cause the growth of other lipomas in other parts of the body. Most lipomas grow individually in various areas of the body. If you have multiple lipomas, then that is another type of lipoma and may not be connected to the single lipoma that appeared in other areas of your body.

There is no need to panic when you see an individual with lipomas. Although lipomas can sometimes be painful especially when they grow relatively large and blocks or presses on nearby nerves, they are not fatal and contagious. Other factors that can trigger this medical condition include injury, trauma or heavy blows to the body because of accidents.

## *Is Lipoma Related To HIV?*

Lipoma is a benign tumor that develops between the skin and the layer of muscles. These benign tumors slowly grows and can even take years before they can increase in size making them quite difficult to diagnose and notice early on. Some people acquire this condition at young age and only notice the lumps when they are already adults when the lumps started to grow relatively bigger enough to be noticed or to cause pain.

HIV on the other hand, is a virus and is one of the most dangerous viruses in the world today. This virus can develop into numerous serious health conditions since the virus mainly attacks the immune system of the body making patients with this virus vulnerable to various types of health problems.

# Useful Websites

## Sites in USA –

http://www.mopical.com/product.html

Here are some sites in Australia, where you can find Lipoma aids –

http://www.mopical.com/-product not scientifically tested, but is being widely used

http://www.naplofax.com/-naturopathic 'product

http://www.lemeton.com/– the Lipoma products available here has not been tested by the FDA. It is made up of natural ingredients. They have a disclaimer that if the product does not work, you should go and talk to your doctor.

http://www.earthclinic.com/CURES/lipoma.html-you are not going to get any products here, but you are going to get a number of useful tips, for natural cures, based on personal experience.

http://www.lipomahelp.org/-gives you information about lipoma products.

http://www.iherb.com/-you can get natural herbs, vitamins and supplements on this site. Is considered to be a really good natural products site.

---

## Websites offering liposuctions in US, Canada, Australia & UK

http://www.liposuction.com/-this site gives you extremely good and detailed information about professional liposuction doctors in your particular state or area.

http://www.lipodoc.com/–affordable liposuction in Chicago.

San Diego liposuction center – http://www.sandiegoliposuctioncenter.com/– affordably priced liposuction center in San Diego.

Lipo sculpting – http://www.lipo-sculpting.com/Orlando-FL/?gclid=CLjR6vbZk54CFQtM2god7FuI6A – liposuction center in Orlando, Florida

Bassin plastic surgery - http://www.bassinplasticsurgery.com/floridasmartlipo.htm?gclid=CNyOnPXZk54CFURR2god8luY6A – has liposuction branches in Melbourne, Florida and Tampa.

Rodeo Drive plastic surgery, Beverly Hills, LA

http://www.rodeodriveplasticsurgery.com/proced-lipo.html?gclid=CMyO5qTck54CFRdc2goduHJI6g

Westlake dermatology – Austin, Texas
http://www.westlakedermatology.com/cosmetic-procedures/plastic-surgery/liposuction-austin-tx/

David B Reath Austin, Texas
http://www.dbreath.com/index.cfm/PageID/102

---

# Canada

http://www.lipo.ca/-this website gives you important information about a number of experienced professional liposuction surgeons in Ontario, BC, Manitoba, Québec, Alberta, New Brunswick and other provinces of Canada.

http://www.findprivateclinics.ca/Liposuction/130-0.html – the site is going to give you plenty of information about private clinics in Canada, where you can get liposuctions done.

http://www.doctorseanrice.com/html/body-liposuction.html – Dr. Sean Rice is the first doctor to offer laser liposuction services in Canada. His services are offered to patients in the GTA area as well as in New York.

http://www.novasans.com/liposuction/canada/- this is a site where you can check prices and different clinics for liposuction procedures.

# Australia

Here are some well-known and popular sites for lipo-suction procedures, in Melbourne, Sydney, Brisbane and Adelaide.

http://www.liposuctionaustralia.com.au/

http://www.cosmosclinic.com.au/

http://www.ashleycentre.com.au/

http://www.paulbelt.com.au/liposuction

http://www.cosmeticmedical.com.au/proc/lipo.html

http://www.drlanzer.com/liposuction

http://www.melbplastsurg.com/html/body.html

http://www.bodyrecon.com/home/liposuction-geelong/
http://www.mrich.com.au/

http://www.whatclinic.com/cosmetic-plastic-surgery/australia/liposuction

http://www.whatclinic.com/cosmetic-plastic-surgery/australia/south-australia/liposuction-the site allows you to compare the services offered to you by 10 clin-ics in South Australia.

# United Kingdom

http://www.whatclinic.com/cosmetic-plastic-surgery/uk/liposuction-this site gives you information about 145 liposuction clinics all over the UK.

Other well-known UK liposuction clinics are given below –

http://www.thecosmeticclinic.com/cosmetic-surgery/liposuction.html

http://www.cadoganclinic.com/liposuction-clinic-london/

http://www.harleybodyclinic.co.uk/

http://www.harleymedical.co.uk/cosmetic-surgery-for-women/the-body/liposuctionfat-removal-liposculpture/

http://www.londonhouse.uk.com/

http://www.dralexchambers.co.uk/fat-removal/vaser-liposuction.html

http://www.mya.co.uk/cosmetic-surgery/liposuction

# References

Kempson RL, Fletcher CDM, Evans HL, Henrickson MR, Sibley RS. Tumors of the Soft Tissues, Atlas of Tumor Pathology, AFIP Third Series, Fascicle 30, 2001

Fletcher CDM, Unni KK, Mertens F. Pathology and Genetics of Tumours of Soft Tissue and Bone, World Health Organization Classification of Tumours 2002

Weiss SW, Goldblum JR. Enzinger and Weiss's Soft Tissue Tumors, 4th edition, 2001

Furlong MA, Fanburg-Smith JC, Childers EL. Lipoma of the oral and maxillofacial region: Site and subclassification of 125 cases. Oral Surg Oral Med Oral Pathol Oral Radiol Endod. 2004 Oct;98(4):441-50.

Dal Cin P, Sciot R, Polito P, Stas M, de Wever I, Cornelis A, Van den Berghe H. Lesions of 13q may occur independently of deletion of 16q in spindle cell/pleomorphic lipomas. Histopathology. 1997 Sep;31(3):222-5.

Rubin BP, Dal Cin P. The genetics of lipomatous tumors. Semin Diagn Pathol. 2001 Nov;18(4):286-93.

Fletcher CD, Akerman M, Dal Cin P, de Wever I, Mandahl N, Mertens F, Mitelman F, Rosai J, Rydholm A, Sciot R, Tallini G, van den Berghe H, van de Ven W, Vanni R, Willen H. Correlation between clinicopathological features and karyotype in lipomatous tumors. A report of 178 cases from the Chromosomes and Morphology (CHAMP) Collaborative Study Group.Am J Pathol. 1996 Feb;148(2):623-30.

Mandahl N, Mertens F, Willen H, Rydholm A, Brosjo O, Mitelman F. A new cytogenetic subgroup in lipomas: loss of chromosome 16 material in spindle cell and pleomorphic lipomas. J Cancer Res Clin Oncol. 1994;120(12):707-11.

Miettinen M, Sarlomo-Rikala M, Kovatich AJ.Cell-type- and tumour-type-related patterns of bcl-2 reactivity in mesenchymal cells and soft tissue tumours. Virchows Arch. 1998 Sep;433(3):255-60.

Horiuchi K, Yabe H, Nishimoto K, Nakamura N, Toyama Y. Intramuscular spindle cell lipoma: Case report and review of the literature. Pathol Int. 2001 Apr;51(4):301-4.

French CA, Mentzel T, Kutzner H, Fletcher CD. Intradermal spindle cell/pleomorphic lipoma: a distinct subset. Am J Dermatopathol. 2000 Dec;22(6):496-502.

Suster S, Fisher C, Moran CA. Expression of bcl-2 oncoprotein in benign and malignant spindle cell tumors of soft tissue, skin, serosal surfaces, and gastrointestinal tract. Am J Surg Pathol. 1998 Jul;22(7):863-72.

Suster S, Fisher C. Immunoreactivity for the human hematopoietic progenitor cell antigen (CD34) in lipomatous tumors.Am J Surg Pathol. 1997 Feb;21(2):195-200.

Templeton SF, Solomon AR Jr. Spindle cell lipoma is strongly CD34 positive. An immunohistochemical study.J Cutan Pathol. 1996 Dec;23(6):546-50.

Zelger BW, Zelger BG, Plorer A, Steiner H, Fritsch PO. Dermal spindle cell lipoma: plexiform and nodular variants. Histopathology. 1995 Dec; 27(6):533-40.

Fanburg-Smith JC, Devaney KO, Miettinen M, Weiss SW. Multiple spindle cell lipomas: a report of 7 familial and 11 nonfamilial cases. Am J Surg Pathol. 1998 Jan;22(1):40-8.

Furlong MA, Fanburg-Smith JC, Miettinen M. The morphologic spectrum of hibernoma: a clinicopathologic study of 170 cases. Am J Surg Pathol. 2001 Jun;25(6):809-14.

Enzinger FM, Harvey DA.Spindle cell lipoma.Cancer. 1975 Nov;36(5):1852-9.

Billings SD, Folpe AL. Diagnostically challenging spindle cell lipomas: a report of 34 "low fat" and "fat-free" variants. Am J Dermatopathol. 2007 Oct;29(5):437-42.

Zamecnik M, Michal M. Angiomatous spindle cell lipoma: Report of three cases with immunohistochemical and ultrastructural study and reappraisal of former 'pseudoangiomatous' variant. Pathol Int. 2007 Jan;57(1):26-31

Hawley IC, Krausz T, Evans DJ, Fletcher CD. Spindle cell lipoma—a pseudoangiomatous variant.Histopathology. 1994 Jun;24(6):565-9.

Diaz-Cascajo C, Borghi S, Weyers W. Fibrous spindle cell lipoma: report of anew variant. Am J Dermatopathol. 2001 Apr; 23(2):112-5.

# Index

## A

adiposis Dolorosa · 22, 52
Adiposis Dolorosa. · 18
alternative · 36, 53, 55, 62, 66, 74, 75, 89
Angliolipoma · 9
apple · 79

## B

biophysiological · 52
breast Lipoma · 15, 16
bulging · xiii

## C

Cancerous · 17
Chondroid lipoma · 11
Complications · vi, vii, 97, 98, 104
complications. · 4, 60, 103, 104

## D

Dercum disease · 23, 24
detoxification · 34, 35, 70, 78
doctors · 18, 47, 51, 58, 71, 104, 107, 112
Dogs · 25, 27, 28

## E

Exercising · 70, 85

## F

facial Lipoma · 15
fatty lumps · 1
Fibrolipoma · iii, 13
fructose corn syrup · 53

## G

genetically · 2, 16, 19, 51, 52, 64, 101

## H

hereditary · 16, 28, 35, 103, 108
hormonal imbalances · 28

## I

injections · 15, 55, 59, 61, 62, 99

## L

Labrador · 26
Lemon juice · 36, 70, 95
liposarcoma · 12, 44, 107
liposuction · 52, 59, 60, 61, 62, 99, 107, 112, 113, 114, 115

## M

Madelung disease · 106
malignant · 12, 19, 46, 47, 48, 118

medication · 6
miraculous pills · 90
mobility · 4, 30, 97
MRI and CT scan · 6
Myelolipoma · iii, 12

## N

Numbness · 65

## O

obese · 21, 27, 101
overweight · 25, 27, 30, 31

## P

physicians · 3, 14, 43
Pleomorphic lipomas · iii, 13
preservatives · 34
protuberant · 40
psychological · 41

## S

spinach · 80
Steroid · 61
surgery · 3, 7, 18, 23, 32, 55, 59, 60, 103, 104, 107, 112, 113, 114, 115

## T

to Xanthoma · 32

tumor · 1, 2, 5, 7, 11, 12, 15, 18, 19, 25, 26, 31, 33, 35, 39, 40, 41, 43, 45, 46, 47, 49, 55, 58, 59, 65, 71, 76, 94, 98, 103, 104, 105, 108, 109
turmeric · 67, 69, 70, 75, 76, 82, 83, 94

# ABOUT THE AUTHOR

There are many treatment guides for lipoma removal out there from dozens of people claiming to be experts. However, very few of these so-called "lipoma treatment experts" practice what they preach or have the credentials to back up their claims. Since you are probably wondering how this program is different, here's the story of Thomas McPherson, the author of this book:

Thomas McPherson has been involved in the alternative health industry researches, for many years. He has keen interest in writing comprehensive treatment guides and alternative health books.

A few years ago, Thomas battled with several lpomas all over his body and he was diagnosed with dercum's disease. He experienced both painless and painful lipomas in many parts of his body including his face and he suffered with all other rear relentless symptoms associated with lipoma: such as burning sensations, intermittent aching pain and low self-esteem from the fatty lumps that disfigured his face.

After he was diagnosed with dercum's disease and was specifically told by several doctors that there wasn't a cure for my condition, he started down the long, frustrating road of trial and error until he finally pieced together a complete and comprehensive method used by thousands of lipoma sufferers to permanently remove their lipomas.

Thomas McPherson spent countless man-hours to study and research the information in this book. He used to spend hours at the library swallowing stacks of books, journals and magazines about lipoma, fatty lumps, cancer, tumors, and other serious skin conditions.

He literally read hundreds of traditional medicine and alternative medicine books from cover to cover on the subject. His library quickly grew to over 279 health and holistic books and he read every word almost to the point of memorizing them.

But he didn't just read. He interviewed countless of other lipoma sufferers and endlessly picked the brains of every doctor, herbalist, homeopath and naturopath kind enough to lend some minutes of their time and fragments of their expertise and knowledge only to find a solid solution that removed his lipomas permanently. This piece of work is his detailed research on the condition.

If you have further question you can reach him on his email:

ThomasMcpherson@LipomaRemovalNow.com